Applauding *Eat Efficiently*

Our bodies are not our own; we were bought with a price. So we must be faithful stewards of God's property.

Madonna Woolford
R.N., B.S.N.

We need to be proactive in health: Mind, Body, Spirit, and Soul.

Debra Griffin Stevens
D.N.P., M.S.N., R.N.C-M.N.N.

During my college years, my eating habits were extremely undisciplined. Through the life-changing information found in this book, my habits now reflect my lifestyle; good health and abundant life.

Dawn Gordon Smith
Wife, Parent, M.Ed – Teaching and Learning

We are all works in progress committed to excellence, as we flow; so we may as well eat healthily as we grow.

1K Phew (Glenn "Isaac" Gordon, II)
Hip-Hop Artist

In life we go from one anxious moment to another. We must stop justifying unhealthy eating habits, then searching for quick fixes to become healthy. This book will assist you with changing your habits, today.

Glenn D. Gordon
B.S. Sociology

Human expression of righteousness is incomplete unless there is focus on sanctifying the body. I am personally encouraged to make the dictums a permanent part of my life. It is my hope that you will do the same.

Anthony Williams
M.D., M.P.H.

HARRIET WEST GORDON

P E E L

EAT EFFICIENTLY

NO BRANCH CAN BEAR FRUIT BY ITSELF;
IT MUST REMAIN ON THE VINE.
JOHN 15:4B

DISCLAIMER

The information presented herein is in no way intended as a substitute for medical counseling. This book was written to provide experiential information. Neither Harriet, Glenn D. Gordon, GHD Inc., nor any member of the organization's board shall have liability or responsibility to any person with respect to damage, injury, or any alleged causes resulting from information in this book.

All scripture quotations, unless otherwise indicated, are from the King James Version of the Holy Bible.

Cover designed by Harriet Gordon, LPC
ISBN: 978-09862166-1-9

GOD'S DIVINE HANDWORK, INC.

Our organization's goal is to affect the lives of people in the communities which we serve. God's Divine Handiwork, Inc. (GHDI), is a family-oriented organization which has deep concern for the well-being of our society. We desire to see people "well" in all aspects of their lives. We aim to educate society regarding academic, spiritual, emotional, and physical health. Conferences, forums, seminars, classes, and workshops may be arranged for your specific needs. Our services include courses entitled, but not limited to:

Healthy Living
Test-Taking Tips
Time Management
Parenting to the End
PEEL, Volume 1: Pray Powerfully
PEEL, Volume 2: Eat Efficiently
PEEL, Volume 3: Exercise Enthusiastically
PEEL, Volume 4: Learn, Laugh, & Live Lovingly
PEEL, Volume 5: Cook Consciously

Contacts us: **peelv5@gmail.com** and on Facebook:
http://www.facebook.com/peelv5

"It's the quality of your days rather than the quantity of your years that really counts.

Enjoy life! "

—*Harriet Gordon, LPC*

DEDICATION

I0100084

PEEL, Volume 2: *Eat Efficiently* is dedicated to the Body of Christ who can live victoriously in every area of life – which includes taking care of your total health and fitness.

To my family who gives me unconditional love and support.

Dedicated to the memory of my father, _Tommy West, Jr_ and his entire family. I love you.

CONTENTS

ACKNOWLEDGEMENTS. 10

FOREWORD 12

PREFACE 15

CHAPTER 1 19

CHAPTER 2 29

CHAPTER 3 36

CHAPTER 4 40

CHAPTER 5 49

CHAPTER 6 59

CHAPTER 7 64

CHAPTER 8 74

CHAPTER 9 81

CHAPTER 10 88

CHAPTER 11 94

CHAPTER 12 97

CONCLUSION 102

REFERENCES 112

ABOUT THE AUTHOR 114

ACKNOWLEDGEMENTS

Thank you for your wealth of expertise while taking care of our family through the years:

Dr. Titus D. Duncan, MD
Surgeon; Atlanta, GA
Dr. Tyrone Malloy, MD
Gynecology and Obstetrics: Decatur, GA
Dr. Fiona Blair, MD
Pediatric Medicine; Stone Mountain, GA
Dr. Anthony Williams, MD
Preventive Family Medicine; Columbus, OH
Dr. James Bennett, MD
Urologist; Atlanta, GA
Dr. Robert Monett
General Family Medicine; Decatur, GA
Dr. Vincent Vaughters, DDS
General Dentistry; Decatur, GA
Dr. Martin Dixon, DO
Family Medicine; Lithonia, GA

My husband, Glenn; son, Isaac; and daughter, Dawn and family.

FOREWARD

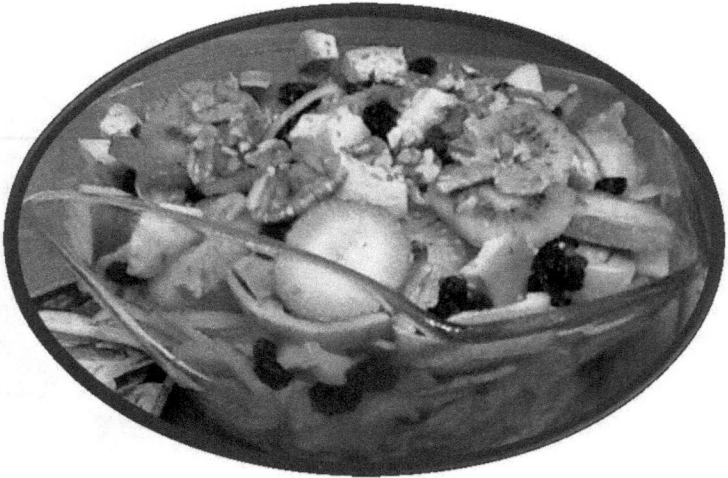

Every day, three hundred and sixty-five days of the year, I take on the responsibility of deciding what my wife Ruth and I will eat and where we will dine. The task is not easy and the choices are numerous. Everywhere you turn there are food choices.

To further complicate the situation, you have the question of "Why do we eat the foods that we do?" Well, there are personal preferences: garlicky, Indian, salty, Chinese, grandma's soul food, or just plain American food (whatever that is). Likewise, we have to deal with tradition, social interactions, convenience, habits and beliefs. However, there is one thing missing from our difficult selections: **Nutrition!!!**

In this book, Deacon Gordon has compiled all the information concerning living in good health. He motivates us to open our minds to facts concerning what is good for us and those things which will cut-off life. This book is designed to help us climb to the highest level physically, emotionally, and spiritually possible.

After reading "Healthy Living", you will understand the essentials of good eating. In fact, you will understand the critical nature of disciplining yourself to proper eating habits.

(The Late) Jimmie Lee Smith, Archbishop Light of the World Christian Tabernacle International

What more noble endeavor can an individual pursue than to improve, tend, maintain and indeed sanctify his or her own physical body which is the earthly temple of the soul? Human expression of righteousness is incomplete unless there is focus on this item of the triune of body, mind and spirit. Just as we feed our minds with the Word of God and nurture our spirit in prayer and meditation, so too must we nourish the physical body with the proper quality and quantity of food and drink.

This book is a wonderful compendium of helpful, facts regarding nutrition, general health and wellness and contains precepts that are easy to read and apply right away. Inspired by his family and chiseled by a life time of trials and challenges, Glenn Gordon has offered all who read his work a fresh and exciting opportunity to learn and grow in health and well-being. I am personally encouraged to make the dictums a permanent part of my life. I hope you will also do the same.

Anthony Williams
M.D., M.P.H.

PREFACE

Community leaders, pastors, families, and individuals who desire to empower others and themselves will be blessed by this book. It is impossible to exude healthy nurturing if you are unhealthy. Proper healthcare can break strongholds in geographical regions and individual lives. Proper nutrition can turn generational curses into generational blessings.

Do you know which foods to eat in order to avoid common diseases or conditions? The resounding reply from most people is "no."

Healthy Living 2nd Edition was prepared with you in mind. Although you are encouraged to read it thoroughly, the chapters have been designed for independent use. This handbook addresses the many "W" questions (who, what, when, where, and why concerning proper nutrition) which were prepared for your journey to a healthier lifestyle.

Our world produces a plethora of healing, nutritious and healthy foods, yet we participate in an enormous amount of artificial flavors, fat, salt and preservatives. In our daily lives, we go from one anxious moment to another. In fact, we justify eating unhealthily for convenient foods which leaves us looking for quick fixes to become healthy, happy, smart and small. We consult with pastors, counselors and physicians to learn of moral character, physical health or justice, often dismissing the most basic rule in life, **"How to Eat."**

Our society pays greatly for our years of excess. Diabetes, cancer, obesity and heart disease are among the high prices we pay. Though many diseases are avoidable, they are now affecting very young children. Where did we go wrong? How can we change our fatal eating habits? We need to slow down long enough to reach for the Holy Bible, the book which has sustained men and women for thousands of years. In it is the real miracle diet, alongside all of God's other miracles.

The Bible illustrates the importance of bread, grains, nuts, fruits, and vegetables. Our society typically consumes these foods but are we preparing them properly? They were created with a purpose and it has been proven that when we do not know the purpose of a thing, we will abuse it. Misuse is abuse. As you read this book, your questions about healthy living are addressed accordingly, you should begin to do your part in contributing to a healthy society. This book includes numerous details for our well-being.

Nuggets for well-being:

- *Sunshine* – 15 minutes in the sun will lower your blood pressure. It also turns your body's cholesterol into Vitamin D. It is free, use it!
- *Water* – Drink lots of it. It will cleanse your body tissues and give you energy.
- *When to Eat* – Eat your largest meal in the morning, a moderate lunch, and sparingly in the evenings. Meals should be spaced 4 to 5 hours apart.
- *When to Drink* – Drink 15 to 20 minutes before meals or two hours after meals. Drink at least 8 glasses of water per day.
- *When to Sleep* – Our bodies heal themselves between 9p.m. and 12

midnight. Every hour of sleep that you get before midnight is worth two hours of sleep that you get after midnight.

The "who, what, when, where, why, and how" of eating a healthy, nutritious and healing diet are important questions which deserve truthful answers. The natural order which God created is marvelous! Why can't we use wisdom with what God has given us? He sent the Israelites food every day during their forty years in the wilderness, and He still provides.

This is the second in a series. For victory in every area of your life, consider the advice from each volume of P.E.E.L.

P.   PRAY POWERFULLY – Vol. 1
E.   EAT EFFICIENTLY – Vol. 2
E.   EXERCISE
       ENTHUSIASTICALLY–
       Vol. 3
L.   LEARN, LAUGH, LIVE
       LOVINGLY – Vol. 4

CHAPTER 1
WHAT'S AILING YOU?

As you read this book, please keep in mind that it is not intended to take the place of medical advice. We strongly encourage you to seek the opinions of medical professionals. The following is a list of foods to aid in improving the conditions which ail you. The results are based on studies conducted by different health institutions and medical schools:

- Spinach may prevent or relieve depression.
- Garlic cloves cut heart attack risk in half.
- Fish oil stunned growth of cancerous colon polyps.
- Fats removed from the male diet strengthened the reproductive organs.
- Oats may help you to stop smoking.

- Soybeans relieve symptoms of menopause.
- Green tea retards artery clogging
- Chili peppers fight colds and congestion better than cold medicines
- Yogurt cuts cold and Hay Fever symptoms.
- Onions may relieve and prevent asthma.
- Avocado may improve cholesterol.
- Removing cow's milk from an infant's diet often cures colic.
- Avoiding mild and cheese may help manage some symptoms of arthritis.

What is ailing you may easily be corrected by changing your eating habits. In cultures where high amounts of fiber are consumed, conditions such as constipation, appendicitis and hemorrhoids are rare. Fiber is the part of fruits, vegetables and grains that your body can't digest. Some fibers remain unchanged as it speeds up your food's trip through your digestive system. Many nutritionists believe you would be healthier with higher amounts of fiber in your diet can help you avoid or deal with conditions in a healthier way.

Conditions Fiber Fights

Diabetes – Fiber helps improve the way your handles insulin and glucose. Eat whole grain rather than refined carbohydrates. Dark rye bread, whole-wheat crackers, multi-grain bagels, and bran muffins are good choices.

Heart attacks and strokes – The fiber in oatmeal, okra, and oranges helps eliminate much of the cholesterol that can clog your arteries, and cause a stroke or heart attack.

Constipation and hemorrhoids – Sweet potatoes, barley, and pinto beans, provide roughage. They keep the stool moist, soft, and easy to eliminate.

Appendicitis – Fruits such as apricots and peaches aid in keeping bowel content soft.

Diverticulosis – Pouches, called diverticula, can cause abdominal pain if they are inflamed. As your body processes fibrous foods like peas, spinach and corn, it tones up your intestinal muscles. No more pain!

Weight gain – Since fiber swells, you will feel satisfied faster. When you have room and desire dessert then you may select fruits like strawberries or plums. Low-fat, low-calorie vegetables and grains are the best foods to eat for losing weight.

Impotence – Beans contain a protein, L-arginine that helps to improve impotency. Zucchini yellow squash, and brussel sprouts are fiber-filled vegetables which help maintain strong blood flow to the penis by lowering your cholesterol and keeping vessels unclogged.

Cancer – An increased amount of fiber in your diet speeds cancer-causing compounds out of the digestive system. The more animal fat in a diet the higher the incidence of bowel cancer has been detected. The more bulky, fiber-rich foods people eat the less unhealthy fat they are likely to eat.

Foods such as whole grains, legumes, fresh fruits and vegetables are natural protectors against gallbladder disease, varicose veins, hiatal hernia and other conditions which ail you. Gradually add fibrous foods to your diet. Adding too much too soon will cause these side effects: gas, bloating, abdominal cramps and diarrhea.

This is a process to consider when adding fiber to your diet:

- **Start the day with a whole-grain cereal.** Add raisins, sliced bananas or chopped apples to a cereal which contains 5 or more grams of fiber per serving.
- **Eat some vegetables raw.** When you cook vegetables, steam them or sautee them until tender. Munch on carrot or celery sticks and lunch on crunchy garden salad.
- **Snack on fresh and dried fruits.** The most fiber is located in the skins of fruits and vegetables; eat the skins.

- **Substitute brown rice for white.** There are less-familiar grains to try; some include kasha, couscous, or bulgar.

- **Add beans to soups and stews.** To prevent gas and bloating, do not cook dried beans in the same water you soak them in. Substitute meat with bean burritos or red beans.

- **Sip some psyllium.** When you do not get enough fiber in your diet, supplement your diet with Metamucil – made from the fiber of ground psyllium seeds. Metamucil helps your bowels function normally.

Is cancer, diabetes, or hypertension really hereditary or are they direct results of our poor
eating habits? Let's look at foods which aid in combating these diseases.

CANCER

Fruit – All fresh fruits are rich in antioxidant vitamins and phytochemicals which are capable of neutralizing carcinogenic (cancer causing) substances entering the body. Lemons, oranges, grapefruits, plums, pineapples, grapes, blackberries, strawberries, blueberries, acerolas, and kiwis are the most effective in cancer prevention.

Olive Oil – This should replace other oils. Olive oil reduces the risk of breast cancer.

Whole Grains – They accelerate movement through the bowel. Whole Grains retain and remove carcinogenic substances that may be in the digestive tract. Fiber in grains and whole-grain breads work best in the prevention of stomach and colon cancer by reducing the time that these harmful substances are in contact with the digestive tract.

Wheat Germ – It stops the processes of cellular degeneration and protects against cancer.

Vegetables – All vegetables aide in the prevention of cancer. The most effective are: red beets, carrots, tomatoes, sweet peppers, eggplant, cabbage, cauliflower, broccoli, and radishes.

Natural Yogurt – Yogurt protects against breast cancer.

Legumes (beans) – Beans are rich in fiber and anti-carcinogenic phytochemicals.

DIABETES

Antioxidants – They are important to help regulate glucose in the blood. Vitamin B group and trace elements should be taken. Trace elements help produce insulin. Antioxidants are found in eggs, fresh fruits, vegetables, wheat germ, and brewer's yeast.

Nuts – Eat oil bearing nuts.

Artichoke – Lowers the level of sugar in the blood.

Celery – Helps regulate blood glucose level, reduces cholesterol and neutralizes excess acids that may be produced in the body because of diabetes.

Avocado – Helps to maintain an adequate blood sugar level.

Onion – Reduces blood glucose.

Potato – Use in controlled amounts. Potatoes release glucose during digestion.

Wheat Germ – Four to five spoonsful may reduce the glucose level and the need for insulin.

Whole Grains – Barley, oats and wheat should be used liberally by diabetics.

Legumes – They regulate the level of glucose in the blood because of their fiber content. Beans should be the fundamental food of a diabetic.

Fruit – Fruit is extremely necessary in cases of diabetes. Mangos and bananas are tolerated best.

Vegetables – All vegetables are tolerated well by diabetics and because of their low calorie content, they help treat the obesity typical of adult diabetics.Recommended vegetables for diabetics are: *broccoli, cabbage, cauliflower, cucumbers, endive, escarole, green beans, lettuce, and peas.*

HYPERTENSION

Animal protein should be avoided during the treatment of hypertension.

If you desire to exercise healing power on the cardiovascular system, eat these foods:

- Beans
- Celery
- Dark Green Leafy Vegetables
- Flaxseed (Ground)
- Garlic

- Grapefruit
- Guava
- Onions
- Pears
- Squash

If you have been diagnosed with hypertension, eliminate these foods completely or use in moderation:

- Alcohol
- Coffee
- Eggs
- Ham
- Matures Cheese
- Meat
- Pepper
- Salt
- Saturated Fat
- Sausage
- Stimulant beverages

Sodium is present in certain foods, additives and medications. Keep your sodium intake between *1250 and 2500mgs per day*. Read the food labels and be sure you are eating foods that may improve or treat conditions which ail you.

CHAPTER 2
WHAT ARE THE
"RIGHT" FOODS?

There is so much confusing information. How do you know if you are choosing the right foods? Many health problems may be prevented when you make the right choices. It is evident that you care about eating nutritious foods. How do you choose the foods to eat? The major factors are:

- Price
- Taste
- Ease of preparation

However, a highly recommended place to start is to use the characteristics below for a healthy diet:

- **Adequacy** - You use up vitamins and minerals, daily. Be sure your diet provides adequate nutrients, minerals, and vitamins.
- **Balance** – Extra nutrients of one source will not make up for too little of a different source.
- **Calorie Control** – Calories you do not burn get stored as fat which can lead to obesity and other health problems.

- **Moderation** – This does not mean total "abstinence". Limit certain foods such as fat, cholesterol and sugar.
- **Variety** – Many foods contain small amounts of toxins and contaminants your body does not notice unless you eat them a lot. Eat plenty of different foods. This process allows you to get all the nutrients you need and enjoy mealtimes more.

Why eat the right foods? It is important to eat the right foods because our bodies do not belong to us. I Corinthians 3:16,17 tells us that we are the temple of God:

"Know ye not that ye are the temple of God, and that the Spirit of God dwelleth in you? If any man defile the temple of God, him shall God destroy; for the temple of God is holy, which temple ye are."

I Corinthians 6: 19,20 says that your body is the temple:

"What? Know ye not that your body is the temple of the Holy Ghost which is in you, which ye have of God, and ye are not your own? For ye are bought with a price: therefore glorify God in your body, and in your spirit, which are God's."

2 Corinthians 6: 15-17 shows us that light has no part with darkness:

"And what concord hath Christ with Belial? Or what part hath he that believeth with an infidel? And what agreement hath the temple of God with idols? For ye are the temple of the living God; as God hath said, I will dwell in them, and walk in them; and I will be their God, and they shall be my people. Wherefore come out from among them, and be ye separate, saith the Lord, and touch not the unclean thing; and I will receive you."

We are only stewards over God's property. It is imperative that we take care of what has been placed in our care as the Lord tells us in **Luke 12:42:**

"And the Lord said, Who then is that faithful and wise steward, whom his Lord shall make ruler over his household, to give them their portion of meat in due season?"

In Luke 16:8 we see the Lord commend the unjust steward for acting in wisdom:

"And the Lord commended the unjust steward, because he had done wisely; for the children of this world are in their generation wiser than the children of light."

The time will come when we will have to give an account of what we have done. Luke 16:1 states:

"And he said also unto his disciples, There was a certain rich man, which had a steward; and the same was accused unto him that he had wasted his goods."

The following eating plan which was designed by nutritionists to show you how food should actually look on your plate:

➤ Vegetables, fruits, whole grains and beans should cover two-thirds or more of the plate. Plant foods lower your risk of many diseases.

➤ Meat, fish, poultry or low-fat dairy foods should cover no more than one-third of the plate. You may mix three ounces of meat or less with grains, veggies or beans.

➤ When selecting healthy foods, pay attention to the calories you take in. Remember to ignore diets which encourage you to cut back on fruits and vegetables. Do not put your long-term health at risk for short-term weight loss. Fad diets with high-protein, low-sugar and low-carbohydrate directives can be confusing when it comes to some basic principles.

➤ You will find it easier to maintain a healthy weight for life once you suit your portions to your needs. However, most people do not really understand how much food is equal to one serving size. One cup is the standard serving of most cereals. What you consider to be one serving is probably closer to two servings. Let's make it easier to remember by comparing it to something familiar:

Raw vegetables	= your fist
Cooked vegetables	= the palm of your hand
Pasta	= one scoop of ice cream
Meat	= a deck of cards
Grilled meat	= a checkbook
Butter, margarine, peanut Butter, or cream cheese	= your thumb first joint
Pretzels or chips	= 1 handful
Chopped fruit	= a tennis ball
Apple	= a baseball
Potato	= a computer mouse
Steamed rice	= a cupcake wrapper

Are you looking for the best eating plan for a long and healthy life? Your plan should meet these three basic requirements: *It should be*

➤ Made up of foods that are easy to digest and eliminate.
➤ Nontoxic.
➤ Provide enough nutrients and fuel to satisfy your daily needs. Moreover, the **right food** is not the only ingredient necessary for a healthy life.

If you desire additional security of a healthy and long life, consider the following plan:

HEALTHY LIVING

- *P.rayE.atEfficientlyE.xerciseL.earntoLaugh*
- *Get sufficient sleep*
- *Limit alcohol*
- *Do not smoke*
- *Begin tasks and appointments on time*
- *Respond to communications*
- *Do not over extend commitments*
- *Avoid using names on answering devices*
- *Buckle your seatbelts*
- *Drive safely*

P.E.E.L. EAT EFFICIENTLY by Glenn D. and Harriet Gordon

CHAPTER 3
WHAT WAS THE "STAFF OF LIFE?"

The "staff of life" during biblical times was wheat. It was such an important part of everyday survival until it became an important religious symbol for both Jews and Christians. The periodic famines were taken to be signs of God's displeasure and the abundance of harvest was His blessing. During these times the people expected to have some type of grain at every meal. For instance, Ezekiel Bread has about every type of grain available as ingredients. **Ezekiel 4:9** says:

"Take for yourself wheat, barley, beans, lentils, millet and spelt and put them into one vessel and make bread of them for yourself."

Let us take a closer look at wheat.

WHEAT
The outermost layer of the wheat kernel is the wheat bran, which is all fiber.
Fiber is critical to healthy digestion and efficient bowel function. Wheat bran is also loaded with Vitamin B and protein.

It is also rich in iron, magnesium, zinc, chromium, manganese and Vitamin E.

White bread has three times less the amount of fiber found in whole wheat bread. Our best protection against and cure for constipation is the fiber in wheat. Bowel functions are improved; intestinal infections, hemorrhoids and varicose veins are prevented.

Doctors stress that anything we can do to minimize bowel and digestive problems deduces the risk of fatal colon cancer from developing.

An attempt to compare the effectiveness of various vegetable fibers as sources of bulk in our diets was demonstrated by a team of researchers.

Subjects for the demonstration were given wheat bran, carrots, cabbage and apples to eat. In conclusion, all the vegetables were useful for various reasons, but none came close to matching the effectiveness of wheat bran.

Gradually increase the amount of wheat fiber in your diet.

Three tablespoons of unprocessed bran per day or one-third of a cup of 100 percent whole-wheat bran cereal is enough for most people. However, if you have a history of chronic constipation, you may require more. The coarser the grain, the better the results will be.

Though the consumption of bran is a cure for constipation, it is only the first of many health benefits offered. The more this cereal-type we eat, the less likely we are to develop bowel and rectal cancer.

In other parts of the world where their fiber consumption is much higher than in the United States, colon and bowel disorders are rare. One example was a study conducted with farmers from Finland. They ate lots of grains which blocked the formation of cancers. The same was true centuries ago in the lands of the Bible where fiber-rich diets; especially grains, were standard fare.

The Bible mentions several types of grains and ways to use them that are as good today as they were centuries ago. Cereals and whole-wheat breads are not the only way to get the fiber you need. Here is a closer look at barley:

BARLEY

A diet which includes barley three times a day, has lowered blood cholesterol by about fifteen percent in a number of medical studies. The same high fiber content keeps us regular, relieves constipation and keeps away a variety of digestive problems.

It also helps block cancer. Barley is effective at shutting down the liver's production of the bad cholesterol that does so much damage to our arteries and can cause strokes and heart attacks.

In one interesting study on animals, it was discovered that the production of bad cholesterol was reduced by eighteen percent when large amounts of barley were added to the animal's diets. A follow-up study was conducted on men. A high barley diet had the same effect on humans. In the study, a group of men ate lots of cereal, bread, cakes, and muffins made from barley flour.

After six weeks of three-a-day servings, the men's cholesterol levels dropped an average of fifteen percent. At the supermarket or health food store, look for the word "unpearled" on the box. That means the barley is unprocessed and higher in fiber, which also helps lower blood pressure.

Food for Thought
Wholesome breads and grains add fiber, which is vital for our digestive health.

CHAPTER 4
WHY DO YOU NEED AN "APPLE A DAY?"

One common activity for a healthy lifestyle is eating an apple a day. Apples are high in fiber, vitamins, minerals and antioxidants. They are fat-free, cholesterol-free and low in sodium. The more this cereal-type we eat, the less likely we are to develop bowel and rectal cancer. The more this cereal-type we eat, the less likely we are to develop bowel and rectal cancer. . The Bible never says what fruit the serpent used to tempt Eve in the Garden of Eden.

Tradition tells that it was an apple; what we do know is that in the Bible, the apple gets high marks for its healthful healing powers. Even modern science has confirmed this.

The apple is credited for improving conditions of gout, rheumatism, jaundice, liver and gallbladder troubles in addition to nervous and skin diseases caused by a sluggish liver and hyperacidity.

Other healing credits of apples:

- ➤ Apples suppress the appetite without robbing the body of necessary nutrients, so they are great for dieters.
- ➤ Natural juices in apples are highly effective virus fighters.
- ➤ They lower both bad cholesterol and high blood pressure.
- ➤ They help stabilize blood sugar; important factor in controlling diabetes.
- ➤ Apples help prevent constipation, or help treat diarrhea.
- ➤ They prevent tooth decay.
- ➤ They contain chemicals that scientists believe are vital in stopping cancer.

According to the editors of F C & A Medical Publishing, apples will keep you healthy for a long time. Listed are a few of the various ways: Apples –

Regulate your day – You do not have to be concerned about being regular anymore. Whether your problem is visiting the bathroom too often or not often enough, apples can help. One apple with its skin contains four to five grams of fiber – the most important nutrient in keeping your bowels working like a well-oiled machine.

Keeping yourself regular without relying on harmful laxatives could be as easy as replacing that afternoon snack of potato

chips or cookies with a crisp, delicious apple. Applesauce is actually the best apple product for diarrhea since it is made without the high-five skin.

Keep your body young – Many diseases that seem to be a part of aging are kept from you by antioxidants. So many people are taking supplements for protection that it has become a multibillion-dollar industry. A fresh apple has more that fifteen times the antioxidants power of the daily recommended dose of vitamin C.

Research also proves that ordinary apples were able to stop the growth of colon and liver cancer cells in test tubes. Unpeeled apples were especially effective. Why purchase additional supplements when you can get better antioxidants firepower from a sweet, crunchy fruit? This is just another "W" question.

Cut your risk of heart disease - Sometimes it is hard to remember which food is good for which part of your body. When you pick up your next apple,

examine it carefully. It is shaped a bit like a heart – and that should help you

remember apples are good for your heart! It is the magnesium and potassium in apples that help regulate your blood pressure and keep your heart beating

steadily. It is a naturally occurring antioxidant, flavonoid quercetin that protects your artery walls from damage and keeps your blood flowing smoothly.

Strike at the heart of strokes – Apples are even a smart choice for helping avoid strokes. The connection is clear – people who regularly eat apples are less likely to have strokes than people who do not.

Protect your joints – Few people get arthritis in areas of the world where fruits and vegetables make up a large part of the diet. Apples contain boron, a trace mineral many plants absorb from the soil. Boron is credited in preventing arthritis. You need
three to ten milligrams a day to affect your risk of arthritis. It is not reasonable to eat nine apples a day. Try pairing an apple with peanut butter, or raisins.

Help you breathe deeply – Air pollution, pollen, cigarette smoke and other air-borne nastiness assault your lungs daily. Besides, you may suffer from asthma, emphysema or a lung condition. Sometimes all you want to do is to take a deep breath. Grab "an apple a day". Unfortunately, apples cannot reverse an existing lung condition, but you can add a line of defense against future damage and alleviate the severity of your symptoms.

When purchasing apples, be sure they are not bruised; they are firm and have good color. At home, take them out of their plastic bag and store them in your refrigerator – loose in the produce bin or in a paper bag are best. Apples absorb odors, so keep them away from strong smelling foods such as garlic or onions. Be careful of purchasing cider from a roadside stand; harmful E.coli bacteria could be present in unpasteurized apple juice or cider. Always try to buy organically grown apples (produced without chemicals). If you can not find organically grown apples, either scrub your produce well or sacrifice that fiber-rich peel before eating.

Other Fruits

Bananas – Aid the muscular and nervous systems – the natural sugars are ready for use as fuel. Also, the banana promotes sleep and contains enzymes that assist in the reproduction of sexual hormones.

Blackberries – Relieve diarrhea; an astringent and a tonic.

Blueberries – Improve sluggish circulation and benefits the eyesight; especially night vision. They may be used in the treatment of varicose veins, hemorrhoids, and peptic ulcers. They rejuvenate the pancreas and aid in relieving dysentery. Fresh berries help heal mouth infections. Blueberries are laxatives and a blood cleanser.

Cherries – Cherries relieve painful urinary infections and stop constant urination. Cherries are well-known remedies for gout, arthritis, and rheumatism. They combat the harmful effects of animal protein, and benefits the liver blood and gallbladder.

Dates – Dates were among the most abundant of all fruit of the Holy Land. These sweet fruits grow on palm trees that can be 100 feet high. They grow in clusters with as many as 200 dates per cluster. They can be yellow, orange, red, green, or brown.

Figs – Have been prized since ancient times for their sweetness and nutritional value. Greek and Roman athletes ate figs to increase their stamina and improve their performance.

Grapes – Grapes with seeds help cut the mucus and catarrh of the body so they can be eliminated. They detoxify the body; especially good for the digestive tract, liver, kidneys and blood. Their simple sugars are absorbed into the bloodstream. Grapes aid in improving anemic conditions.

Grapefruit – Aids in the removal or dissolving of inorganic calcium which may have formed deposits in the joints (arthritis
for example). It normalizes red blood cells levels. Excellent for the cardiovascular
system; helping to lower blood cholesterol. It is a natural antiseptic for wounds and is
valuable as a drug or poison eliminator.

Lemon – Nourishes the brain and nerve cells. It reduces fevers, destroys putrefactive bacteria in the intestines and mouth and alleviates flatulence and indigestion. Strengthens the body structures and makes for healthy teeth. May be used as a hair rinse or facial astringent.

Melon – (Cantaloupe)- Cleanses and rehydrates the body. Rejuvenates and alkalinizes the body. It is used in patients with heart disease to keep the blood thin and to relieve angina attacks; requires no digestion when eaten alone.

Orange – Daily use will aid in toning up and purifying the entire system. Aids digestion and stimulates the activity of the glands in the stomach.

Raspberries - Are beneficial for all female organs, they help relieve menstrual cramps, and will decrease the menstrual flow. Good cleanser for mucus and for toxins in the body.

Strawberries – Good for the intestinal tract; a cleansing food that rids the blood of harmful toxins. If you rub a clean cut strawberry over the face, it will clear the skin.

Watermelon – Alleviates stress and depression. It is a cooling food, and an excellent / detoxifier for the entire body. It is a diuretic. The white rind of the melon is one of the highest organic sodium foods. The outer peel is one of the best sources of chlorophyll. As a diuretic, it quickly flushes the bladder.

Food for Thought
A variety of fruits and vegetables provide the basis of good nutrition.

CHAPTER 5
WHEN SHOULD YOU EAT VEGETABLES?

In recipes, some vegetables are extremely versatile when used to flavor other dishes. They are delicate and form the basis of many traditional dishes which originated in ancient Israel and neighboring lands. The Bible says that in the earliest days of creation, all of God's creation, even animals were vegetarians. As you read, you will find out when to eat which vegetables and what God designed it to do.

Asparagus – Neutralizes excess amounts of ammonia in the body and aids in preventing the rupturing of small blood vessels. Asparagus encourages evacuation of bowels by increasing fecal bulk with undigested fiber. It serves as a blood builder due to its chlorophyll content and contains many of the elements that build the liver, kidneys, skin, ligaments and bones.

Avocado – Regulates the body functions and stimulates growth. It aids in red blood regeneration and prevention of nutritional anemia. When used regularly, it will improve hair and skin quality as well as soothe the digestive tract. It contains organic fat and protein.

Broccoli – Contains almost as much calcium as whole milk. Benefits rough skin and counteracts the sulphur compounds
that form gas.

Brussel Sprouts – Stimulates the liver and other tissues out of stagnancy. They are rich in alkalizing elements with specific affinity for the pancreas. Aids in reducing the risk of cancer; especially colon cancer.

Cabbage* – Detoxifies the stomach and upper bowels of waste; therefore, improving digestive efficiency and facilitating rapid elimination. Works to alkalize the body, stimulate the immune system, kill harmful bacteria and viruses, soothe and heal ulcers, reduce the risk of cancer, and clear up the complexion. It also improves blood circulation.

Carrots – Nourish and stimulate almost every system in the body. Help kidney function, reduce the risk of cancer, balance the endocrine and adrenal systems and depress blood cholesterol. Carrots are beneficial for the eyes and vision. They kill parasites and unhealthy intestinal bacteria and increase bulk elimination from the colon.

Cauliflower – If eaten raw, cauliflower aids bleeding gums and helps to purify the blood. It is helpful in improving the conditions of asthma, kidney and bladder disorders, high blood pressure, and constipation. Cauliflower should not be combined with other high sulfur content food.

Celery – Tones the vascular system, lowers blood pressure and may be useful in case of migraines. Stops the digestive fermentation of foods, purifies the bloodstream, aids digestion and helps clear up skin problems. Celery dislodges calcium deposits from joints and holds them in solution until they can be eliminated through the kidneys. Helps repair damaged ligaments and bones.

Collards – These dark green leafy vegetables have anti-cancer antioxidants properties. They mildly stimulate the liver and other tissues out of stagnancy.

Corn – Corn on the cob is high in fiber. Yellow corn is helpful in building bone and muscle and is an excellent food for the brain and nervous system. It is the easiest of all grains to digest.

Cucumber – Helps dissolve uric acid accumulations such as kidney and bladder stones. It destroys worms, especially tapeworms. Good for both high and low blood pressure.

Leeks – Have been prescribed for infertile women and were used internally and externally for a variety of conditions including obesity, kidney complaints, intestinal disorders and coughs.

Lettuce – Has large organic water content. Helps renew joints, bones, arteries and all connective tissue. Helps cure insomnia and nightmares.

Mushrooms – They help lower the risk of cancer, thin the blood – lowering cholesterol and aid in preventing strokes
and heart attacks. Mushrooms stimulate the immune system, increase oxygen efficiency, counteract the effects of pollutants and increase resistance to disease.

Onions – During the Bible days, onions were used to treat colds and similar conditions. They block the viruses that cause colds and stimulate the body to produce more fluids, which in turn loosen mucus and make it easier to cough up. There are 150 chemicals in onions, and the sulfur in onion works well in stopping cancer cells.

Onions block sudden increases in blood sugar and help to control diabetes. They are effective against several
dangerous bacteria including the E.coli and salmonella. Onions kill bacteria responsible for illnesses ranging from diarrhea to tuberculosis.

Peppers – Peppers and chilies boost the secretion of saliva and stomach acids, increase peristaltic movement and feed the cell structure of the arteries, veins, and capillaries. Make body tissues more resistant to colds; promote growth and the feeling of well-being. Aid in food absorption and normalize the brain and nervous system. Chili peppers are excellent for clearing sinuses.

Potato – Contains a sugary carbohydrate which is readily digested and enters the bloodstream slowly to provide the constant
energy we need; excellent fuel food. Potatoes are useful to those who use too much salt and high sodium foods in their diets.

Spinach – Helps build healthy blood; valuable for the eyes. Provides organic mineral salts required for repair and maintenance of the colon. Detoxifies the digestive tract and soothes intestinal inflammation. Spinach serves as a laxative.

Sweet Potato – Easily digestible and good for the elimination system, ulcers, inflamed colon and those with poor circulation. Sweet Potato can bind heavy metals by sticking to the objects and pulling them out. They are very nutritious.

Tomato – A natural antiseptic. Tomatoes are effective in reducing liver inflammation due to hepatitis and cirrhosis.

Now, the benefits of legumes.

LEGUMES (or Bean)

Beans are in the legume family and are high in protein. They are packed with fiber to keep you regular and to keep your cholesterol and blood sugar down. You can reduce the amount of gas they produce by changing the water while they boil. Also, you may use "Beano" by adding a few drops after cooking to make your beans *wind-free*. Beans have a number of healthy benefits:

Flush out cholesterol – Fiber works as a bouncer for cholesterol particles. The particles get shown to the door before they can do any damage.

Increase blood flow – The protein L-arginine is in beans. It can increase blood flow. Add a few servings and see if you notice a difference.

Cut your cancer risk – What you eat could be a life or death decision. Chemical substances in beans called lignans and phytochemicals are natural cancer fighters.

Olive (oil) The use of high levels of olive oil offers substantially reduced risks against heart attacks and strokes. It is rich in monounsaturated fats which may lower

blood cholesterol. Four to five tablespoons of olive oil daily dramatically improve the blood profiles of heart attack patients. Two-thirds of a tablespoon daily lowered blood pressure in men.

Olive oil also blocks the growth of cancer cells. Olive oil is rich in vitamin E, one of the best antioxidants available. Experts believe that those antioxidants help human cells fight off cancer. In doing so, they fortify the cells and slow down deterioration that accompanies the aging process, since the cells are healthier and live longer.

Olive oil has a number of uses:

> Hair　　　　Mix with egg yolk and lemon juice; rub on hair; rinse after 5 minutes.

> Dandruff　　Mix with cologne; rub into scalp and hair; rinse after 5 minutes.

> Dry Skin　　Mix with avocado; mask the face; rinse after 10 minutes.

> Wrinkles　　Mix with lemon juice; rub into the skin at bedtime.

> Soft Skin　　Mix with salt; massage well; rinse with cool water.

> Strong Nails Soak nails in warm oil for 5 minutes; pat nails with white iodine.

> Feet　　　　Massage for rejuvenation.

> ➤ Muscles   Mix with rosemary; massage into muscles where achy.

> ➤ Complexion Mix equal parts with lavender oil; massage face.

> ➤ Lower   24 olive leaves; 8oz water; Boil 15 minutes; Cool; Blood   Pressure Drink morning and night.**(has   slight laxative effect)

Reducing the Risk for Viruses

Recipe for Stir Fry Cabbage /Ingredients:

1 Green cabbage - medium
Bell peppers – 1yellow; 1red
Carrots/shred-sliced – 2 cups
1 Yellow onion – large
1 Garlic clove – small
Cut of chili pepper – small (optional)
Olive oil – 1 tablespoon
Lemon pepper – dash
Sea Salt - dash (optional)

Needed: 1Large Deep Frying Skillet with lid; Medium Spatula; Sautee to Frying at high Temperatures

Directions:

Prepare vegetables by cleaning and washing. Then, thin slice bell peppers, onions, and cabbage to desired size. Thin slice carrots; mince chili pepper and garlic.

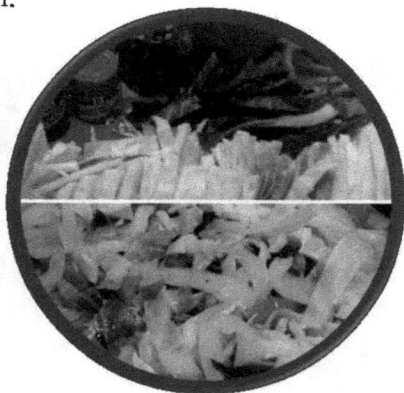

Prepare a large skillet:Completely cover the bottom of the skillet with olive oil, liberally to prevent the veggies from sticking; Place the skillet over heat; slowly add one veggie at a time (bell peppers, onion, carrots, cabbage, garlic, chili pepper) – using the wooden spatula to stir and turn as veggies sautee. Cover with lid and reduce heat.

Steam for six minutes; Drain (if desired); Season to taste!

Harriet W. Gordon- @1/2004

CHAPTER 6
WHAT ARE THE CAUSES OF COMMON DISEASES?

Our environment contains numerous conditions or diseases that may be prevented. If we would become much more cautious concerning what goes into our systems, we would live healthier, happier and longer lives.

Following is a discussion of the common causes of this culture's conditions and diseases. Research proves that prevention will take place when people pay attention to their root causes. This discussion is listed alphabetically and no other hierarchy is intended:

Allergy – The physical discomfort or irritation due to excessive retention of waste in the system when food is eaten which has the effect of stirring up toxins in the body.

Anemia – Deficiency of red blood corpuscles or of the red coloring matter of the blood, caused by prolonged habit of eating foods in which the calcium and other atoms have been devitalized, such as canned foods, starches, and pasteurized milk.

Angina – Occurs with pain around the central chest area, often triggered by overeating and indigestion.

Arthritis – Inorganic calcium deposits in the cartilage of the joints, as a result of eating concentrated carbohydrates in excess.

Asthma – Extreme difficulty in breathing due to mucous accumulation in the bronchial tubes.

Astigmatism – A dysfunction in vision due to the imperfect condition of the eye as a result of organic atoms lacking in the nourishment of the optic system, accentuated by the presence of waste matter in the organs and glands directly affecting the eyes. The thyroid, liver, gall bladder, pancreas and colon are all glands and organs whose inefficient operation is a direct contributing factor in any dysfunction of the optic system.

Blood Presssure (High) – The result of impurities in the blood vessels caused by the build up of deposits in the blood stream of inorganic atoms accumulating from cooked and processed foods (particularly concentrated starches and sugars) and by retention of waste in the eliminative organs and channels.

Blood Pressure (Low) – Primarily due to nutritional deficiency as a result of eating all or mostly cooked and processed foods.

Brain Tumors – The result of defective cells invading the surrounding tissues; they form tumors.

Bronchitis – Inflammation of the bronchial tubes due to excessive mucus in the system.

Cancers – Defective cells and improper digestion; especially in the digestive system.

Cirrhosis of the Liver – The direct effect of overworking the liver as a result of eating too many starches (particularly white flour) causes the liver tissues to harden.

Constipation – A colon filled with toxins resulting in hard or difficult to pass stools. This may result from unhealthy eating habits.

Cramps – Pains due to the presence of the gas resulting from foods improperly combined.

Decay (bone) – The decomposition of bone tissue is due to excessive use of milk and concentrated starches.

Decay (tooth) –The decomposition teeth of bone tissue is due to excessive use of milk and concentrated starches.

Diabetes – The inability of the pancreas to metabolize carbohydrate due to excessive use of concentrated starches and sugars in the diet.

Diarrhea – Is nature's way of cleansing the colon.

Eczema – The inflammatory condition of the skin due to excessive acidity of the lymph glands and the elimination through the pores of the skin of waste matter, which should really pass out through the kidneys and the bowels.

Epilepsy – The nervous spasm resulting from excessive toxemia and starvation of
the nervous system. It is sometimes caused by the presence of worms in the colon.

Fatigue – Is an indication that the cells of the body are not getting sufficient live atoms in the food to furnish the constant flow of new energy needed.

Gout (Rheumatism) – Caused by the inflammation of the ligaments of a joint, bone or lining due to the overproduction or insufficient elimination of uric acid.

Halitosis – Results from the retention of fermented and putrefied food wasted in the body.

Hay Fever – May be caused by excessive use of milk, starches and grain products.

Headaches – This is a signal that the body is overloaded.

Heart Trouble – Caused when cholesterol clogs the blood vessels, preventing an adequate flow of blood.

Hemorrhoids – A direct result of putting bowel muscles under too much strain.

Leukemia – Is caused by insufficient organic atoms in the diet; too much cooked food, starches, sugars and meats.

Migraine – Results from impure blood stream and improperly nourished nerve centers.

Multiple Sclerosis – The brain stems are attacked and are unable to control movement.

Prostate Trouble – Enlargement of the prostate obstructs the free flowing of urine from the bladder.

Tumors – Are growths due to a lack of sufficient organic elements and caused by the excessive use of concentrated inorganic foods, mostly flour products.

Varicose Veins – The results of blood valves becoming weak and leaking. The valves collect blood and bulge.

Food for Thought

Herbs and spices add flavor to meals and help fight a host of ailments.

CHAPTER 7
WHY EXERCISE?

There are four basic ingredients that are necessary in order for the body to sustain physical life. They are:

> ➤ Oxygen (air)
> ➤ Water
> ➤ Food
> ➤ Exercise

Food is the least important of these basic needs, as you can usually live past 40 days without food. Without water you can not live more than four days. Without air you can not live more than four minutes. However, without motion the body cells will slowly die!

The body needs physical activity because the tissue cells, of which the body is composed require daily stimulation to maintain their elasticity and pliability. They will become weak, sickly and begin to malfunction if they are not exercised on a regular basis. Cells will cease to function if they continue to go without exercise.

A person who exercises vigorously on a regular basis will experience fewer health problems than the person who does not exercise. Additionally, the person who exercises removes the toxins and debris
from the system. Without daily exercise, tissue cells hose their elasticity. If the body
does not receive a sufficient supply of oxygen, people become forgetful and eventually senile. According to a study by the National Academy of Sciences' Institute of Medicine, Cognitive decline is not inevitable. A study of what *helps* and what *hurts* cognitive functioning was included. Highlights from their study are discussed by Elizabeth Agnvail:

WHAT HELPS
Exercise – Aerobic exercise is especially beneficial for brain health, and even better when combined with strength training. Exercising for at least thirty minutes or
more at a time appears to be better for brain health than shorter sessions.

Remaining socially and intellectually active – Activities that challenge your brain – including reading books, writing letters, and learning a new language – all help preserve brain function. So do social activities such as volunteering, playing cards, attending worship services, and talking to friends.

Eating a balanced diet – Although no specific diet has been proven to maintain or improve brain health, studies of the Mediterranean and DASH (Dietary Approaches to Stop Hypertension) diets justify eating less meat and consuming more nuts, beans, whole grains, vegetables and olive oil. Fatty Acids, as in Salmon, have been shown to help cognition in some studies, though not in others.

Getting good sleep – Poor sleep patterns and quality are linked to cognitive impairment and Alzheimer's. Breathing disorders, such as sleep apnea, also put older people at higher risk for memory problems and dementia.

Keeping your heart healthy – What's good for your heart is also good for your brain. High blood pressure, high cholesterol and diabetes – especially in midlife – are linked to poor brain health later in life. Lowering blood pressure with medication seems to help prevent brain problems.

WHAT HURTS

Depression – In midlife, depression doubles the risk for cognitive decline and dementia, possibly because depression causes changes in the hippocampus. Late-life depression is also linked to dementia; especially vascular dementia, although it's unclear whether the depression may be an early symptom of undiagnosed brain health problems.

Hearing and vision loss – Problems hearing and seeing are both linked to trouble with thinking, memory and
socialization, and should be corrected, when possible. Older adults with hearing problems appear to have a greater rate of brain shrinkage as they age.

Certain medications – Anticholinergic drugs have been shown to increase the risk of dementia – these include antihistamines (Benadryl, sleep meds, antidepressants). Watch out and be aware of side effects.

Stress – Not only can daily stress cause memory problems, but long-term stress is connected with faster rates of decline in brain health, too. Methods to reduce stress (meditation and prayer) may help.

Air pollution – It may be that pollution increases heart disease, stroke and lung problems, which in turn cause problems with brain health. Or that small particles in the pollution directly harm the brain. One new study found that long-term exposure to air pollution is linked with brain shrinkage, brain damage and impaired function.

Without exercise the muscles begin to decrease in size or waste away. You can feel this when you try to use muscles that have not been exercised for a while. Above all, the most important muscle is the heart muscle. When the heart is not exercised, it starts to function improperly, arteries clog, strokes and heart attacks may result. When people suddenly exert an unexercised heart, death can occur. Mowing the lawn with force and shoveling snow are two examples that may cause sudden exertion.

Emotional Health

Physical health is extremely important but it is very important that we do not neglect our emotional health. It has been proven that exercise aids in the prevention of depression. Emotional problems are sicknesses that many deny. When they are recognized, it is often the symptom rather than the cause that is addressed. How many people do you know who are really happy and vibrant? The Lord wants us to be happy: **John 10:10** *"I am come that they might have life, and that they might have it more abundantly."*

Feelings stimulated by the mental or physical parts of our body are our emotions. If we were to keep track of one another's emotions and placed them in two columns, one column would outweigh the other. Our emotions deeply affect our lives and the lives of those around us. All emotions are *positive* or *negative*.

Positive Emotions – Which happens first, the positive emotion producing a healthy body, or a healthy body producing a healthy positive mind? A healthy body has a positive effect on our whole being. When we feel joy, love, happiness, peace or contentment there is a surge of pleasure throughout the body and it emanates to those around us.

Negative Emotions – Negative emotions take energy from the body and hinder the body from cleansing and healing itself. Stress produces more negative emotions when the body is not able to cleanse itself. A person experiences negative emotions when his or her body does not function properly; whether it is due to lack of exercise, a headache, cold, etc. Some emotions send strong waves throughout the body. Additionally, the emotions of fear, worry, sorrow, hate, jealously or anger send negative vibes to others.

Man was created to be physically active. Yet, many people still ask, "Why do I need to exercise?" We exercise because it was on of God's commands:

"And the LORD God took the man, and put him into the garden of Eden to dress it and to keep it". Genesis 2:15

We exercise because the body can not function properly without it. The final and one of the most important reasons is to set a good example for all who are watching you.

We must keep the next generation in mind in all that we do. Children have bodies that are hungry for oxygen, hydration and proper nourishment.

What about the children?

When children are involved, use an increased amount of stimulating movement for proper exercise. Exercise
may come in the form of music, rhythm, rhyme, rap, drama, charades, role-play or dance; however, children need more than occasional exercise. What children need is good balanced nutrition. The nervous system needs these materials for proper functioning. They are proteins, carbohydrates and fats. When we eat foods high in sugars instead of these raw materials needed by the body, the body's ability to protect and restore itself is weakened. Children need raw materials for healthy bodies.

Proteins – The diets of children with learning difficulties usually show a deficiency in protein. Proteins and fats are the major building blocks for membranes
in our body. They are essential for appropriate nerve transmission and development. We need a diet that includes all ten amino acids needed for the synthesis of proteins. Children need extra protein as they form 90% of their nerve cells before the age of five.

Carbohydrates – These consist of the long molecular chains of sugars that provide the main source of energy for the body. Carbohydrates are found in grains, fruits, vegetables and dairy sugar. Carbohydrate intake should be balanced with fats and proteins.

Fats – Fats work as the lubricants for our joints and bones. Fats help cushion our internal organs and regulate body temperature.

Sugars – *Simple* **sugar should be decreased or eliminated from children's diets.** Sugars in our diet contribute to the cycles of stress and disease. Adrenaline may be increased which can lead to a depressed immune system and an increase in infections. These conditions decrease the brain's ability to stay focused, alert and learn at its highest potential.

Nutritional Tips

➤ **Exercise**
➤ **Limit or eliminate fast foods.**
➤ **Avoid unhealthy vending machines.**
➤ **Children need 40 ounces of water daily (use water bottles for**
➤ **measure).**
➤ **Eliminate soft drinks; especially diet drinks.**
➤ **Eat broccoli and red grapes.**

- ➢ **Get rid of coffee, tea and impure chocolate to avoid dehydration.**
- ➢ **Sleep for eight or more hours each night.**

Studies indicate that proper nutrition aids in keeping people alert and contributes to their ability to remain focused. Therefore, certain foods may contribute to children learning at their highest potential:

Sample Brain Food

Eggs	Apples	Broccoli
Beef Liver	Bananas	Dried Beans
Fish	Grapes	Leafy Veggie
Lean Meats	Orange Juice	Boiled Eggs
Breads	Pure Water	Tuna
Tofu	Pears	Whole Grain
Turkey	Wheat Germ	Nuts
Carbos	White Meat	Complex
Yogurt		

CHAPTER 8
WHAT'S AGE GOT TO DO WITH IT?

It is inevitable that if you live long enough, your body will go through significant chemical changes. The ages vary depending on your genes or gender. For men, the age ranges from 40 to 60. But there is good news for men! With proper nutrition and a healthy lifestyle, transitional age related issues and conditions may be alleviated. On the other hand, the "change of life" will occur in women. However, proper nutrition can keep women feeling well and happy during this time.

MENOPAUSE

The end of menstruation or menopause, takes place for most women by age 50. Women may experience this change earlier if you smoke, or later depending on your genes. When the ovaries stop producing eggs each month and menstruation has been absent for one year, it is time for menopause. It may occur at once, as it does when ovaries are surgically removed, or more gradually over several years.

Some women hardly notice a difference during this time, while others have hot flashes, vaginal dryness, indigestion, loss of sleep, depression and mood swings. Most of these unpleasant side effects can be traced to plummeting hormone levels; especially estrogen. Additionally, once estrogen production tapers off, you are at greater risk of heart disease and osteoporosis. Estrogen dramatically lowers bad cholesterol levels and increases your good cholesterol. Also, estrogen helps your body absorb calcium and kills off some of the cells in your skeleton whose job it is to break down your bones.

Treating the Causes

Phytoestrogens – Eating plant foods with phytoestrogens can give you some of the protective benefits of estrogen. Sources are oats, wheat, corn, apples, almonds, cashews and peanuts. Isoflavones and phytoestrogens are found mostly in soy-based foods like soybeans, tofu, miso and soy nuts.

Calcium – Your body needs calcium to keep your bones strong and to avoid osteoporosis. Calcium may help with hot flashes. Sources of calcium are yogurt, cabbage, spinach, molasses, legumes (beans), seeds, and almonds. Drink juices fortified with calcium.

Vitamin E – (as always, consult your healthcare physician before making changes to your diet) Vitamin E counterattacks the threat of postmenopausal heart disease. It fights potential cancer causing substances and keeps blood cholesterol from damaging your arteries. Good sources of Vitamin E are: nuts, seeds, creamy salad dressings, mayonnaise, and avocados. It is a good idea to cut down on other fats when you add more Vitamin E to your diet because these oily substances will cause weight gain.

Helpful Hints

When approaching and during menopause, eat these foods: oats, corn, skim milk, Chinese cabbage, wheat, apples, wheat germ, almonds and peanuts.

Try to avoid foods high in saturated fat; such as red meat. You are also encouraged to avoid alcohol. Remember, too much salt in your diet will make you feel bloated and might make hot flashes worse. In addition, excess salt is not good for your heart and can contribute to bone loss. If you crave salt, try using different herbs and spices on your food instead. Drink lots of water; water keeps your internal organs and your skin in good shape while it flushes extra salt out of your body.

PROSTATE HEALTH

Obviously, preventing prostate problems is the best solution and the right foods can provide some natural help. This male gland is located below the bladder and wraps around the urethra, the tube which carries urine out of the body. This location contributes to the problems the prostate can cause. The general categories of prostate problems are:

Prostatitis – Acute prostatitis causes fever, chills and pain between your legs and in your lower back. Antibiotic treatment usually clears it up. Chronic prostatitis is an infection which returns repeatedly. The symptoms are similar to acute prostatitis, except no fever is present and the symptoms tend to be milder. Bacteria may not be the cause, making it more difficult to treat.

Enlarged Prostate – Half of all men between the ages of 40 and 60 are affected by this common condition. It can cause urinary problems such as frequent urination, difficulty urinating or dribbling. Treatment includes surgery, heat or freezing therapy and laser therapy.

Prostate Cancer – The most common form of cancer among men is prostate cancer and is second only to lung cancer. Early stages of prostate cancer may not

cause any symptoms, so regular screenings are encouraged. Annual screenings are recommended for men over 40.

Treating the Causes

Lycopene – Eating ten servings of tomato products weekly could dramatically cut the risk of prostate cancer. Lycopene, a carotenoid that gives tomatoes their brilliant red color, is probably responsible for this protective effect. Processed tomato products may be more beneficial than fresh tomatoes because, chopping and cooking the tomatoes break down cell walls and then the lycopene is absorbed into the body.

Sources of Lycopene: tomato sauce, ketchup, watermelon, pink grapefruit and guava

Vitamin E – Men are five times less likely to develop prostate cancer when they have high levels of gamma-tocopherol, a form of Vitamin E.

Sources of Vitamin E: seed and vegetable oils, nuts, green leafy vegetables and whole grains.

Zinc – Zinc may shrink an enlarged prostate or reduce the inflammation of chronic prostatitis.

Sources of Zinc: pumpkin seeds, oysters, shellfish, chicken, legumes (beans) and whole grains.

Vitamin D – Doctor's advice is needed when using supplements; high doses may be toxic.

Sources of Vitamin D: sunshine, fortified cereals or dairy foods.

Soy and Green Tea – Studies show that men who drank soy milk at least once a day were 70% less likely to develop prostate cancer. Also, studies show that the polyphenol in green tea when combined with genistein, a substance found in soy, halted the growth of prostate cancer cells.

Garlic – Garlic contains strong cancer protection. It is loaded with antioxidants and other substances which act as boosters to the immune system and protect against cancer.

Cruciferous Vegetables – Eat three servings of these veggies weekly and you could cut your risk of prostate cancer in half.

Sources of Cruciferous Vegetables: broccoli, cauliflower and brussel sprouts.

Helpful Hints

To help prevent prostate problems eat tomatoes, oysters, wheat germ, pink grapefruit, garlic, pumpkin seeks, watermelon, soybeans, green tea and broccoli. Avoid foods which are high in saturated fat, such as red meat and whole-milk dairy products.

If you are a "couch potato", you could be encouraging cancer to invade your prostate as you munch chips and watch television. A high-fat diet and sedentary lifestyle increases your risk of prostate cancer. Monounsaturated fats (olive, canola and peanut oils) may help lower the risk of prostate cancer.

Food for Thought

Fresh fish and low-fat poultry are wonderful sources of protein.

CHAPTER 9
WHAT DO VITAMINS AND MINERALS DO?

When it comes to total health, vitamins and minerals are more precious than silver or gold. They carry life-giving tasks and are extremely unique. When you shortchange yourself, you put yourself in danger. Missing your daily dosage once in a while does not hurt. Just remember, your body needs a certain amount each day.

VITAMINS

Every day, bodily functions like digestion and thinking would be critical without vitamins. Some vitamins act as antioxidants. Without enough of them, your body can not complete major tasks. Antioxidant vitamins come to your rescue by giving up electrons to stabilize free radicals and help keep your body healthy. Vitamins that you can not afford to miss are:

Vitamin A – This vitamin is most for protecting your eyesight but, Vitamin A has many other jobs. It keeps you healthy by assuring that your cells divide properly into new cells. It is involved with vision, growth, bone and tooth development, skin cells and the lining of your digestive system. *Sources of Vitamin A*: liver, dairy products and eggs.

Vitamin B – These vitamins help you fight off sickness and disease. Though each one is important for its own special reason, these nutrients generally help your body carry out its day-to-day chores.

> - **B1** – Turns food into energy and stabilizes the nervous system
> - **B2** – Forms pigments in the retina and prepares the body to confront stress.
> - **B6** – Metabolizes proteins, carbohydrates and fats; produces energy within the cells of the nervous system. Necessary for blood formation.
> - **B3** – Produces energy and builds DNA.
> - **B5** – Produces energy.
> - **B12** – Makes red blood cells, delivers oxygen to the body and aids

the formation of substances to protect the nerve fibers.

Sources of Vitamin B: whole grains, nuts, legumes (beans), dairy, dark leafy greens, fish, seeds, cereals, liver and egg yolks.

Vitamin C – This vitamin strengthens capillary and arterial walls and supports your bones and teeth. Vitamin C may be the most popular vitamin of all. Well known as a cold cure; a cancer fighter and the king of antioxidants. It deserves all the attention it gets. It is a safeguard from free radicals and it is also in charge of making collagen. Collagen assists in holding together all the cells and tissues of your body, including ligaments, tendons and scar tissue.

Sources of Vitamin C: citrus fruits and bright colored fruits and veggies.

Vitamin D – Helps to build bones, controls calcium and phosphorus levels in your body.
Sources of Vitamin D: fortified milk, eggs, liver and sardines.

Vitamin E – Protects the cells and prolongs their life span. It neutralizes the harmful effect of free radicals. Facilitates the activity of other antioxidants, provides protection against cancer and is involved in the formation of spermatozoids and ova.

Sources of Vitamin E: vegetable oils, dark leafy greens, nuts, seeds and wheat germ.

Vitamin K – This vitamin aids in forming blood clots and controlling calcium levels.

Sources of Vitamin K: dark leafy green vegetables.

MINERALS

If you could remove all your body's minerals and place them on a scale, they would weigh about 5 pounds. Approximately 4 pounds would be *calcium* and *phosphorus*.

Calcium- This mandatory mineral aids in bone and tooth formation, muscular contractions, nerve impulse transmission and blood coagulation. Small amounts of calcium travel to your blood. It regulates blood pressure and keeps the heart muscle pumping.

Sources of Calcium: small bony fish and legumes(beans).

Phosphorus – It is involved in the chemical reaction that releases energy. Phosphorus works hand in hand with calcium to build and maintain strong bones
and teeth. It also helps to turn food into energy. *Sources of Phosphorus:* meats and dairy products.

Chloride – Chloride helps all body cells get nutrition, and it is the main ingredient in stomach acid.
Sources of Chloride: salt (in moderation)

Magnesium – It helps keep your bones and teeth healthy, then it makes sure calcium, potassium, Vitamin D and proteins do their jobs. After you flex your muscles, it is magnesium which helps them to relax. Magnesium deficiency could increase your risk of heart attack and high blood pressure.
Sources of Magnesium: nuts, legumes(beans), whole grains, dark leafy greens and seafood.

Potassium – Keeping blood pressure regulated, maintaining heartbeat, balancing water in cells, secreting insulin in the pancreas, and helping muscles and nerves work properly are a few of potassium's many important jobs. Like magnesium, potassium is beneficial to heart health.
Sources of Potassium: fresh fruits and veggies, fish and legumes(beans).

Sodium – The body needs sodium to maintain its balance of fluids; however, if you do not limit your intake of sodium or salt, you put yourself at risk of heart disease.

Sources of Sodium: Limit your salt and processed foods.

Sulfur – This mineral is especially important in proteins because it gives them shape and durability. Your body's toughest proteins – hair, nails and skin have the highest amounts of sulfur.

Sources of Sulfur: protein-packed foods.

Iron – Is helpful in the formation of hemoglobin of the red blood cells and cellular respiration.

Sources of Iron: meats, eggs, legumes and dried fruits.

Zinc – It helps to maintain skin, hair and nails. Zinc is beneficial in the development of the reproductive organs.

Sources of Zinc: meats, legumes (beans) and whole grains.

WATER

Water cushioned your entire body against the shocks of the world before you were born. Today, it only cushions your joints and spinal

Glenn D. and Harriet West Gordon

column.   Water helps regulate your body temperature, lubricates your digestive tract and maintains pressure in your eyes.   Why drink between eight to twelve cups of fluids per day?

Replenish your supply. You need to drink as much liquid every day as you lose through perspiration and excretion. Otherwise, your body will become

dehydrated. If you lose five percent of your body fluids and do not replenish them, you may experience headache, fatigue, lack of concentration and an elevated heart rate. Lose greater amounts and you face the risk of confusion, shock, seizures, coma and even death.

Sip water during the day. Do not wait until you feel thirsty to drink a glass of water. Your thirst, especially as you get older, may not be a reliable gauge of your body's need. You could be two cups before you feel it.

Drink more when it is hot. You will need more water when you get more exercise than usual or when the weather is hot and dry. Eating plenty of juicy fruits and

veggies or soups may require you to drink less water. When you want something other than water, natural juices and herbal teas are good substitutes.

CHAPTER 10
WHICH FOODS ARE HIGHER IN SODIUM?

Studies have found that people with the highest intake of salt are twice as likely to develop health problems (including cataracts) as those getting low salt intake.   Being aware of the sodium content of selected foods, should help you to reduce your sodium intake.

For a healthier lifestyle, try herbs instead of salt to spice up your favorite foods. Treat yourself to an herbal dish and you might get favor with your lenses. Try these cooking herbs or seasonings:

Parsley – Parsley contains a substance that prevents the multiplication of tumor cells. It relieves gas, stimulates normal activity of the digestive system and freshens the breath. It helps bladder, kidney, liver, lung, stomach and thyroid functions.   Good for high blood *pressure and indigestion.*

Uses for Parsley: vegetables, main dishes, soups, salads and breath freshener.

Sage – One of the most valued herbs of antiquity, sage is highly antiseptic, excellent remedy for colds, fevers, sore throats, relieves tonsillitis, bronchitis, asthma and sinusitis. It has a tonic effect upon the female reproductive reproductive tract;

also estrogenic and is excellent for menopausal problems. It helps to reduce the harmful effects of free radicals.

Uses for Sage: vegetables, soups, main dishes, breads, quiches, scrambled tofu and gravies

Rosemary – Rosemary contains oils which are antiseptic, with antibacterial and antifungal properties which enhance the function of the immune system. By increasing circulation to the skin, Rosemary causes sweating and makes a good remedy to bring down fevers. It stimulates digestion, relieves gas and stimulates liver and gallbladder functions. It is a powerful antioxidant.

Uses for Rosemary: cornbread dressing, vegetables and soups

Thyme – A powerful antiseptic. It enhances the immune system's fight against bacterial, viral and fungal infections, especially in the respiratory, digestive and genitourinary system; such as colds, coughs, flu, gastroenteritis, candida and cystitis.

It has a relaxing effect on the bronchial tubes and acts as an expectorant by increasing the production of fluid mucous and shifting phlegm. Thyme is a liver tonic, stimulating the digestive system.

Uses for Thyme: vegetables, bread, main dishes, soups, rice dishes, pastas, salads and gravies

Garlic – Garlic is an effective remedy against bacterial, fungal, viral and parasitic infections. It contains many sulfur compounds which give it its healing properties. Garlic contains the substance allicin which has been shown to be more powerful than penicillin and tetracycline. It detoxifies the body and protects against infection by enhancing the immune function. It lowers blood pressure and blood levels and improves circulation. Helps treat arteriosclerosis, arthritis, asthma, cancer, circulatory conditions, colds, flu, digestive problems, sinusitis and yeast infections.

Uses for Garlic: vegetables, soups, salads, main dishes, scrambled tofu and as a medicine tea

Dill – Dill has an antispasmodic action, relieving spasm in the digestive tract. It enhances digestion, relieves indigestion, nausea, constipation and hiccoughs. It induces sleep in babies and children, increases milk supply in breast-feeding mothers and relieves painful periods. Dill can be used externally in warming linaments to increase circulation in the limbs and to sooth muscular tension and joint pain.

Uses for Dill: vegetables, soups, breads, and salad dressings

Peppermint – Antibacterial, antiparasitic, antifungal, antiviral and a decongestant. It induces heat and causes sweating and relieves stuffiness. It is a good general tonic that has an excellent cooling effect. Good local application to relieve pain-inflamed joints in arthritis / gout or headache.

Uses for Peppermint: salads, dressings, fruits, beverages and medicine teas

Sodium Content of Selected Foods

Food Item   Amount

- Soy Sauce   1Tbs 1319mg
- Dill Pickles   1 large 1928mg
- Olives-medium   10   258mg
- Catsup   1Tbs   156mg
- Mustard   1tsp   63mg
- Thousand Island Dressing
                           1Tbs 112mg
- French Dressing   1Tbs 219mg
- Italian Dressing   1Tbs 140mg
- Blue Cheese Dressing 1Tbs 164mg
- Mayonnaise   1Tbs   84mg
- Bologna   1 slice 369mg
- Bacon   2 slices 153mg
- Canned Ham   1 ounce 280mg
- Hot Dogs   1 495-627mg
- Corned Beef   1 ounce 282mg
- Sausage Link   1 210mg
- Sauerkraut   1 cup 1755mg
- Pretzels   10 thin 101-200mg
- Cream of Mushroom Soup-can
                           1 cup 1039mg

- ➤ Vegetarian Vegetable Soup-can 1
  1 cup 838mg
- ➤ Bouillon-can   1 cup 782mg
- ➤ Spaghetti Sauce   ½ cup 992mg
- ➤ Cheddar Cheese 1 ounce 198mg
- ➤ Cottage Cheese   1 cup 515mg
- ➤ Buttermilk   1 cup 319mg
- ➤ Tomato Juice   1 cup 364mg

CHAPTER 11
WHAT HAPPENS WHEN SUGAR TURNS SOUR?

We often treat ourselves to sugar, sometimes a double fudge sundae with nuts, holiday candies or homemade pound cake. Because it tastes so good you may not be aware of what it does to your body once it gets inside.

Effects of too much sugar:

Too much sugar depletes the body of Vitamin B and the B Vitamins are essential for healthy nerves. A depletion of B vitamins lowers our resistance to infection
and makes us irritable and depressed.

Too much sugar increases the blood fat levels and tends to clog the arteries. This lowers the body's resistance to diseases. Sugar plays a significant role in the building of cholesterol.

Too much sugar contributes to tooth decay because it slows the fluid flow through the tiny canals of the teeth. The teeth lose their resistance to viral and bacterial invasion and decay results.

Too much sugar weakens the white blood cells which furnish our mainline of defense against invading germs. One white cell can normally attack and destroy 14 invading germs. After eating an excess amount of sugar, this capability is reduced dramatically.

Rich heavy desserts cause irritation of the stomach, mental dullness and obesity. Natural sweets may satisfy the "sweet tooth" while furnishing vitamins and minerals. *Glucose*, natural sugar, is a very basic and necessary food; however, when it is heat processed it changes into an unnatural sugar, *sucrose*. Sucrose leaches vitamin B from the body, destroys calcium, shatters the nervous system, causes teeth to decay, hair to fall out, senility, heart trouble and circulation problems.

When sugar affects your health or turns sour, there are healthy alternatives you may substitute. Please consider making the following changes in your diet, today:

Healthy Alternatives versus Common Sweets

Fruit Sauce vs Syrup
Smoothies vs Ice Cream
Fruit Spreads vs Jams
Water vs Soft Drinks
Dried Fruit vs Candy
Fruit Breads vs Pastries
Wholesome Cookies vs Cookies

Ginger

Take advantage of ginger's powders or toss some chopped ginger into a dish or steep some in a pot of tea. Eat candied or pickled ginger or by the handful.

Some benefits of Ginger: neutralizes nausea, combats cancer, aids digestion, tames arthritis pain, enhances blood flow and soothes heartburn.

Food for Thought

Natural sweeteners, like honey and fruit, are better for us than processed sugars.

CHAPTER 12
FASTING

So much emphasis is placed on the physical exercise and proper eating until we are beginning to examine our lifestyles. Consequently, many people are out of balance by neglecting the spiritual man. The Lord desires order in our lives. We can not serve the Lord to the fullest if our bodies are not functioning as God designed them to function. We can not break God's laws of health and not suffer the consequences. The spiritual man should always be given top priority. Its influence over the physical man is greater than the
physical man's influence over the spiritual. We need proper balance between neglecting our bodies and giving them too much attention.

Therefore, it is appropriate in a discussion for Eating Efficiently, to discuss voluntarily afflicting or disciplining one's flesh, or fasting. The Bible clearly outlines the right way to fast in **Isaiah 58: 6,7**:

> **"Is not this the fast that I have chosen? To loose the bands of wickedness, to undo the heavy burdens, and to let the oppressed**

go free, and that ye break every yoke? Is it not to deal thy bread to the hungry, and that thou bring the poor that are cast out to thy house? When thou seest the naked, that thou cover him; and that thou hide not thyself from thine own flesh?"

Fasting is done by disciplining the flesh while introducing to it a temporary or on-going spiritual discipline.

If you have not fasted before or you are presently experiencing health problems, consult your doctor before beginning a fast. When you have serious concerns or questions, always address them to your healthcare personnel before changing your lifestyle. The way you begin your fast will determine your success. Here are a few suggestions:

> **Have a goal.** Why are you fasting? Is it for spiritual renewal, for guidance, for healing, for the resolution of problems, for special grace to handle a difficult situation?

> **Prepare yourself spiritually.** The foundation of fasting and prayer is

repentance. As you begin your fast, confess every sin that the Holy Spirit calls to your remembrance. Include obvious sins and those that may not be so obvious. God requires us to repent of our sins before He hears our prayers.

➢ **Prepare yourself physically.** You are planning to go without food so you will find it helpful to begin by eating smaller meals before you abstain altogether. This sends your mind a signal that you have entered the time of the fast and it helps to shrink your stomach and appetite.

➢ **Ask for God's guidance.** What type of fast? Does He want you to have only water? Is He asking you to fast one meal per day, one day per week, or several days or weeks at a time? Is God leading you to undertake a forty-day fast? Once you know how to fast, short fasts of one to three days require no more than water. People who fast regularly, often go ten days or longer with beneficial results.

➤ **Limit physical activity.** Exercise moderately. Rest as much as your schedule allows. Short naps are helpful. Your body needs rest from the processes involved in digestion and the assimilation of food to concentrate on excretion.

➤ **Plan prayer time.** Set aside enough time for the Lord. When you pray, fellowship, worship and adore Him the greater your effectiveness and them more meaningful your fast will be. Daily, before leaving home, seek God as you meditate on His Word. There is no set formula for how to pray when you fast. Pray for the fulfillment of the Great Commission.

➤ **End the fast.** When your appointed time of fasting is finished, begin to eat again.

Gradually, reintroduce your stomach to liquids, then soft foods and then solids. It is wise to end your fast with soup. It should be thin, yet nourishing. Then advance to heavier foods. When you fast and pray, expect results! You will feel refreshed as you begin to see results in the situation that originally caused you to fast.

I encourage you to continue to fast and pray until you truly experience victory in every area of your life: physically, socially, academically, emotionally, and especially spiritually. Please pray for youth, couples, families, the church, nation, and the world.

CONCLUSION

MAKE HEALTHY FOOD CHOICES NOW; BE JOYFUL LATER

Years of excess may cause one to pay great dividends. In fact, we justify eating unhealthy for convenience. These products leave us looking for quick fixes to become healthy, happy, smart, or small. There are a number of nutritious and healing foods, yet we choose artificial flavors, fats, salts, and preservatives. Eat a well-balanced diet and learn what you need to *let go* of in life. Do not wait for a near tragic event to occur before you begin eating efficiently. One of my physicians concluded that my healthy diet, not only improved my health and lifestyle, but saved my life!

Create menus which are rich in fruits, vegetables, whole grain and fiber; yet, low in cholesterol and fat. Following is a segment of the lifestyle process which I incorporated:

Efficient Habits:

Sleep – Our bodies heal themselves between 9:00p.m and 12' midnight. Every hour of sleep that you get before midnight is worth two hours of sleep that you get after midnight.

Meals – Eat your largest meal in the morning, a moderate lunch, and sparingly in the evenings. Meals should be spaced 4 or 5 hours apart.

Liquids – Drink 15 to 20 minutes before meals, or two hours after meals.

Water – Drink at least 8 glasses of water per day. It will cleanse your body tissues and give you energy.

Sunshine – 15 minutes in the sun will lower your blood pressure. It also turns your body's cholesterol into Vitamin D. It is free, use it! (Consult your physician for before using supplements).

Making Efficient and Healthy Choices:

Many health problems may be prevented when you make healthy choices for the foods that you eat. Eating properly is important because our bodies do not belong to us. We are the temple of God. Therefore, we must take care of what has been placed in our care. Often, we allow price, taste, or ease of preparation to guide us in our choices. However, using the healthy diet characteristics is the wise place to begin:

Adequacy – vitamins and minerals are used up daily. Be sure your diet provides adequate nutrients, minerals, and vitamins.

Balance – extra nutrients of one source will not make up for too little of a different source. Vegetables, fruits, whole grains and beans should cover two-thirds or more of the plate. Plant foods lower your risk of many diseases. Meat, fish, poultry, or low-fat dairy foods should cover no more than one-third of the plate. You may mix three ounces of meat or less with grains, veggies or beans.

Calorie Control – calories you do not burn get stored as fat which can lead to obesity and other health problems. When selecting healthy foods, pay attention to the calories you take in. Remember to ignore diets

which encourage you to cut back on fruits

and vegetables. Do not put your long-term health at risk for short-term weight loss.

Fad diets with high-protein, low-sugar, and low-carbohydrate directives can be confusing when it comes to some basic principles. You will find it easier to maintain a healthy weight for life once you suit your portions to your needs. Most people do not really understand how much food is equal to one serving size. One cup is the standard serving of most cereals. What you consider to be one serving is probably closer to two servings.

Variety – many foods contain small amounts of toxins and contaminants your body does not notice unless you eat them a

lot. Eat different foods. That way you get all the nutrients you need and enjoy mealtimes!

Fruit and Vegetables

When purchasing fruit; especially apples, be sure they are not bruised, but firm and have natural color. Fruit can absorb odors so keep it away from strong smelling foods; such as garlic or onions. Try to purchase organically grown fruit. If not, be sure to scrub your produce well or sacrifice fiber and *peel* before eating.

Reasons to eat more fruit:

Banana – Promotes sleep and the natural sugars are ready for use as fuel.

Blueberry – Rejuvenates. Has been used as a laxative, and improves sluggish conditions.

Cherry – Combats gout and promotes a healthy urinary tract.

Dates – Serves as a natural laxative with an excellent source of fiber.

Figs – Known to improve performance and increase stamina.

Grapes – Aids in health of digestive tract, liver, kidneys, and blood.

Grapefruit – Improves the cardiovascular system, removes calcium deposits, and lowers cholesterol.

Lemon – Nourishes brain and nerve cells.

Melon – Rehydrates the body.

Orange – Aids digestion, and stimulates stomach activity.

Raspberry – Relieves mucus and toxins in the body.

Strawberry – Rids the blood of harmful toxins.

Watermelon – Detoxifies and washes out the bladder.

Reasons to eat more vegetables:

With regular consumption, you may make these observations-

Asparagus – Contains many elements that build the liver, kidneys, skin, ligaments, and bones.

Avocado – Improves hair and skin quality.

Broccoli – Provides calcium and improves skin.

Brussel Sprouts – Aids in reducing cancer risks.

Cabbage – Improves blood circulation.

Carrots – Beneficial for eyes and vision; may kill unhealthy bacteria.

Cauliflower – Improves conditions of bladder and kidneys.

Celery – Aids in digestions and tones the vascular system.

Collards – Contains antioxidants and stimulates the liver.

Corn – Builds bone and muscle; excellent for brain and nervous system.

Cucumber – Helps to dissolve kidney and bladder stones.

Leeks – Associated with infertility, obesity, and intestinal disorders.

Lettuce – Associated with curing insomnia and nightmares.

Mushrooms – Increase oxygen; aids in reducing risks for strokes and heart attacks.

Olive Oil – Rich in vitamin E which helps cells fight cancer. Cells are fortified and slows deterioration.

Onions – Kills bacteria responsible for illnesses.

Peppers – Makes body tissue more resistant to colds; aids in normalizing the brain and nervous system. Excellent way to clear sinuses!

Spinach – May serve as a laxative; detoxifies the digestive tract and soothes inflammation,

Tomato – Reduces inflammation of the liver.

Eat efficiently and keep the next generation in mind in all that you do. When we eat foods high in sugars, instead of raw materials needed by the body, the body's ability to protect and restore itself is weakened. Efficient nutrition may aid in alertness and contributes to the ability to remain focused. Therefore, by eating certain foods, you contribute to your ability to learn at your highest potential.

EAT YOUR WAY TO EXCELLENT HEALTH

ELIMINATE. When you eliminate all hate, jealousy, impurity, and dishonesty, you have a clean mind that delivers spiritual, mental, and physical force.

ENVISION. Each day, practice healthy visualization. See every organ of your body as performing in the perfect manner for which it was designed. Thank God for your good heart, your good stomach, your good lungs, and for everything given you by God.

EXPECT. The mental attitude profoundly determines the physical condition. To stimulate good health, expect good health, expect vitality, expect vigor, and expect wellbeing.

Key to Successful Health

R.E.S.T.

R READ
RELAXED — Read daily and Bedtime by 11:30 p.m.

E EXERCISE
EFFICIENTLY — Proper nutrition, manage your time, and get appropriate physical activity.

S SAFEGUARD
STUDIES — Study the Bible, get a prayer partner, use Social Media to Send encouragement, and Safeguard your gates: don't allow foul to enter your eyes, ears, nose, or mouth gates.

T TAKE TIME
to TALK — Talk to God, use positive affirmations, and talk with loved ones, daily. :)

Harriet West Gordon   www.facebook.com/peelv5

REFERENCES

Duyff, Roberta Larson, American Dietetic Association's COMPLETE FOOD AND NUTRITION GUIDE, 2nd Edition, Hoboken, New Jersey: John

Wiley & Sons, Inc. 2002.

Editors of FC&A Medical Publishing, *Eat and Heal*, Peachtree City, GA: Frank W.

Cawood & Associates, Inc., 2001.

Green-Goodman, Donna, *Somethin' to Shout About*, USA: Orion Enterprises, 1999.

Lifestyle Principles, Inc., Decatur, GA

Light of the World Christian Tabernacle, International, Stockbridge, GA

Light of the World Christian Tabernacle, *The Power of Fasting*, Stockbridge, GA

Malkmus, George H., Dr, *Why Christians Get Sick*, Shippensburg, PA: Destiny

Image Publishers, Inc. 1997.

Murray, Michael T., *The Complete Book of Juices*, Roseville, CA: Prima Publishing, 1998.

Rivers, Charmaine, *Manna from Heaven*, Boca Raton, FL: Globe Digest Series, American Media Mini Mags, Inc. 2002.

The Internet Explorer, World Wide Web (www.)

Videos: "A Diet for All Reasons," "Diseases Don't Just Happen," "Let's

Eat for Strength."

The Holy Bible: *God's Word*

ABOUT THE AUTHORS

GLENN D. and HARRIET WEST GORDON

are gifted teachers who are dedicated to a *lifetime* of serving. They have passionately and successfully served in ministry roles helping others for over 35 years. They were wed in September of 1978 and are honored parents of two off springs who are also gifted servants: Glenn I. Gordon (Hip Hop Artist; Writer-Producer), and Dawn G. Smith (Choreographer-Dancer; Teacher).

Glenn is deeply concerned for the community and holds a bachelor's degree in Sociology from Wilberforce University in Ohio. Additionally, Glenn has been consecrated for service as a Deacon and a Vocalist; he uses his gifts in God's Kingdom. He is a Community Codes Enforcement Officer, formerly with the city of Atlanta and now serves in Lithonia; DeKalb County, GA.

Glenn enjoys family time, supporting sporting events, and coaching youth team sports. He is an amateur golfer, and is an avid proponent of health and fitness.

Harriet adores family life and nature. She is an education and fitness advocate with more than 35 years of experience. She has received numerous awards for designing and leading transformational train-the-trainer developmental practices. Harriet is an *Intentional* Intercessor, and advisor to parents, youth and young adults.

She gives and donates extra time in areas of research on Aging, Attention Deficit Hyperactivity Disorder (ADHD), Teen Violence, Cancer Awareness, and various intervention / prevention studies. Harriet's passion for family and all humanity leads her to *work* as a sworn Voters' Registrar; and she holds certified licenses in three professions: as a Georgia *Ordained Minister, Counselor, and Teacher.*

This is the power couple's third professional publication. Get prepared to enjoy more fruit from their labor.

Notes:

www.ingramcontent.com/pod-product-compliance
Lightning Source LLC
Chambersburg PA
CBHW071137280326
41935CB00010B/1257